Florence Nightingale Biography For Kids

Inspiring Tales of The Lady with the Lamp, Founder of Modern Nursing, Her Compassion, and Pioneering Spirit for Young Readers Who Love Science and History

Academic Press

1

Table of Contents

1. Introduction

Imagine a dark night in the Crimean War, where wounded soldiers lie in agony, waiting for help. A faint light appears in the distance, moving closer and closer. It is the light of a lamp, carried by a woman in a long dress and a veil. She is Florence Nightingale, the Lady with the Lamp, who has come to offer comfort and care to the suffering men.

But how did this woman become the icon of nursing and healthcare? What motivated her to leave behind a privileged life in England and travel to a foreign land, where disease and death were rampant? What challenges did she face in pursuing her passion and fulfilling her purpose?

To answer these questions, we need to go back to the beginning of her story, to the early years of her life. Florence Nightingale was born on May 12, 1820, in Florence, Italy, to a wealthy and influential family. She was named after the city of her birth, which reflected her parents' love of travel and culture. She grew up in a time when women were expected to marry well and devote themselves to their husbands and children. But Florence had other aspirations. She felt a calling to serve God and humanity, especially the poor and the sick. She was fascinated by mathematics, statistics, and science, and wanted to learn more about the world and its problems. She was determined to make a difference, even if it meant defying the norms and expectations of her society.

This introduction sets the stage for Florence Nightingale's remarkable journey, from a young girl with a vision to a legendary leader of nursing and healthcare. It invites the reader to step into the world of 19th-century medicine, where Florence Nightingale revolutionized the practice and profession of nursing, and improved the health and well-being of millions of people. It also creates a sense of curiosity and anticipation, as the reader wonders how Florence Nightingale overcame the obstacles and challenges that she faced, and what legacy she left behind for the future generations.

2. Early Life

Florence Nightingale's early life was marked by a restless spirit, a thirst for knowledge, and a desire to make a difference in the world. She was born on May 12, 1820, in Florence, Italy, where her parents were enjoying a long honeymoon. She was named after the city of her birth, which reflected her parents' love of travel and culture. She had an older sister, Parthenope, who was named after a Greek island.

Florence grew up in a wealthy and privileged family, who owned two large estates in England: Lea Hurst in Derbyshire and Embley Park in Hampshire. Her father, William Nightingale, was a well-educated and liberal-minded man, who inherited his fortune from his uncle. He was interested in politics, philosophy, and literature, and he encouraged his daughters to pursue their intellectual interests. He taught them several languages, history, and mathematics at home. Florence was a bright and curious child, who excelled in her studies. She also enjoyed reading, writing, and drawing. She had a natural talent for statistics, which she would later use to improve health care.

Florence's mother, Frances Nightingale, was a socialite and a hostess, who came from a family of merchants. She was proud of her status and her connections, and she wanted her daughters to marry well and have a respectable life in society. She was often frustrated by Florence's lack of interest in social events and conventional activities. She tried to mold her into a proper lady, but Florence resisted her mother's expectations. She preferred to spend her time helping the poor and the sick in the villages near her family's estates. She felt a strong sense of compassion and duty, and she believed that God had a special purpose for her life.

Florence's childhood was also influenced by her religious beliefs. She was raised in the Church of England, but she was exposed to different faiths and denominations through her travels and her father's friends. She developed a personal and mystical relationship with God, and she often prayed and meditated. She had a vision when she was 16 years old, in which she felt that God was calling her to do something great. She did not know what it was, but she was determined to find out. She wrote in her diary: "God spoke to me and called me to His service."

Florence's education was unconventional and challenging. She wanted to learn more about nursing, medicine, and health, but these subjects were not considered suitable for women at that time. She faced opposition and ridicule from her family, friends, and society, who thought that nursing was a lowly and menial occupation. She also had to overcome her own doubts and fears, as she struggled with depression and anxiety. She suffered from chronic illnesses and headaches, which affected her physical and mental health.

Despite these difficulties, Florence persevered and pursued her passion. She read books and journals on nursing and health, and she visited hospitals and infirmaries whenever she could. She also sought mentors and teachers who could guide her and support her. She met Elizabeth Fry, a Quaker reformer who improved the conditions of prisons and workhouses. She also met Sidney Herbert, a politician and a friend of her father, who shared her interest in social reform and public health. He would later become her ally and patron in her nursing career.

Florence's most significant educational experience was her training at the Lutheran Hospital of Pastor Fliedner in Kaiserwerth, Germany. She enrolled there in 1844, after her parents finally gave their consent. She spent four months learning the basic skills and principles of nursing, such as hygiene, nutrition, and patient care. She also observed the role and the influence of the deaconesses, who were women who dedicated their lives to serving the sick and the needy. Florence was impressed by their work and their spirit, and she wrote: "It is the training, not the money, that makes the good nurse."

Florence Nightingale's early life shaped her character and her destiny. She was a woman of courage, intelligence, and compassion, who defied the norms and the expectations of her society. She was a visionary, a pioneer, and a leader, who transformed the practice and the profession of nursing. She was a humanitarian, a reformer, and a hero, who improved the health and the well-being of millions of people. She was Florence Nightingale, the Lady with the Lamp, who answered God's call and followed her heart.

3. The Call to Nursing

- Florence's Passion for Helping Others

Florence Nightingale's unwavering dedication to alleviating suffering wasn't forged overnight. It was a flame nurtured from the embers of her childhood, kindled by pivotal moments, and fueled by a relentless inner drive to make a difference.

Early Flickers of Care:

A Tender Heart: Even as a young girl, Florence displayed an innate empathy for those less fortunate. She would tend to injured animals, organize care packages for the poor, and spend hours reading to the bedridden in her village. These acts, though seemingly small, revealed the depth of her compassionate spirit.

Rebellion with a Cause: In her teenage years, Florence's compassion morphed into a desire for systemic change. She defied societal expectations, rejecting a comfortable life of leisure to pursue nursing, a profession deemed unsuitable for women of her class. This act of defiance was the first spark of a lifelong dedication to challenging the status quo and improving the lives of others.

Kindling the Flame:

The Sickbed Revelation: At 17, Florence experienced a personal illness that confined her to bed for months. This enforced stillness allowed her to reflect on the inequalities she witnessed around her. It was during this time that she developed a newfound appreciation for the power of care and the importance of alleviating suffering.

A Walk Amongst the Suffering: In 1849, Florence visited the slums of London. The abject poverty and despair she encountered there left a lasting impression on her. This firsthand exposure to human suffering became a catalyst for her unwavering commitment to improving the lives of the most vulnerable.

Passion in Action:

The Crimean War: During the Crimean War, Florence famously served as a nurse in Scutari, Turkey. Appalled by the deplorable conditions and high mortality rates in the military hospitals, she tirelessly implemented sanitation practices, improved patient care, and advocated for better supplies. Her unwavering dedication saved countless lives and earned her the moniker "The Lady with the Lamp."

[Image of Florence Nightingale tending to wounded soldiers in Scutari]

Beyond the Battlefield: Florence's passion for helping others extended far beyond the battlefield. She established the Nightingale Training School, revolutionizing nursing education and setting new standards for patient care. She also tirelessly campaigned for public health reforms, advocating for improvements in sanitation and hygiene in hospitals and communities.

The Enduring Legacy:

Florence Nightingale's passion for helping others wasn't a fleeting emotion; it was the driving force behind her extraordinary life. It was this unwavering commitment that transformed her from a young girl with a kind heart into a pioneer of modern nursing and a tireless advocate for social change. The legacy of her compassion continues to inspire nurses and healthcare professionals around the world, reminding us that even the smallest acts of care can make a profound difference in the lives of others.

Florence Nightingale's story is a testament to the power of compassion. It reminds us that within each of us lies the potential to make a difference, to alleviate suffering, and to leave the world a little better than we found it. By igniting the embers of our own compassion, we can honor the legacy of Florence Nightingale and continue her vital work in the world.

- Decision to Pursue Nursing

Imagine a vibrant young woman, Florence Nightingale, standing at a crossroads. Behind her lies a path paved with societal expectations – drawing-room soirées, advantageous marriages, and a life of comfortable leisure. Before her, stretches a different route, shrouded in uncertainty – the uncharted territory of nursing, a profession deemed unsuitable for a lady of her standing. This was the defining moment in Florence's life, the critical juncture where she chose to defy convention and chase the calling that tugged at her soul.

The Flickering Flame of Passion:

Florence's path toward this monumental decision was paved with experiences that ignited a passion for caregiving. From tending to injured animals as a child to visiting the impoverished slums of London, she witnessed suffering firsthand. These encounters nurtured a deep empathy within her, a burning desire to alleviate the pain of others.

Internal Conflict and Societal Hurdles:

Choosing nursing meant defying the rigid expectations of Victorian society. Her family, particularly her mother, vehemently opposed her decision. The notion of a young woman of their social standing venturing into the grimy realm of hospitals, surrounded by illness and death, was simply unthinkable. Florence faced societal scorn, whispers of disapproval, and attempts to dissuade her from this radical path.

A Crucible of Conviction:

Yet, Florence remained resolute. Driven by a potent mix of compassion, intellectual curiosity, and a fierce spirit of independence, she refused to be swayed. She devoured medical texts, shadowed surgeons, and even snuck into the local poorhouse to gain practical experience. This clandestine education, fueled by unwavering determination, solidified her resolve.

The Moment of Choice:

Finally, in 1844, at the tender age of 31, Florence made her defining decision. She defied familial disapproval and social censure, enrolling in nursing training at the Institution of Kaiserswerth in Germany. This act of rebellion wasn't just about pursuing a career; it was about claiming her agency, choosing a path that aligned with her deepest values and burning passion.

The Echo of a Choice:

This choice at the crossroads wasn't simply a turning point in Florence's life; it was a pivotal moment in the history of nursing. Her unwavering dedication to this calling transformed the profession, elevating its standards and paving the way for future generations of nurses.

A Legacy Forged in Courage:

Florence Nightingale's decision at the crossroads wasn't just an act of defiance; it was an act of courage, a testament to the power of unwavering passion. It was a choice that redefined the very meaning of womanhood, demonstrating that compassion and a desire to serve could transcend societal limitations. The ripples of her decision continue to be felt today, inspiring nurses and healthcare professionals around the world to follow their calling and make a difference in the lives of others.

Florence Nightingale's story is a reminder that when faced with critical choices, it is the courage to follow our passions, the flame of empathy burning within us, that lights the way to extraordinary journeys. We may encounter crossroads in our own lives, moments where societal expectations clash with our inner calling. But in remembering Florence's unwavering spirit, we can find the strength to choose our own path, the path that leads us towards fulfilling our true purpose and making a lasting impact on the world.

4. Training and Challenges

- Florence's Nursing Training

She felt a calling to nursing from a young age, but her parents opposed her ambition, as nursing was considered a lowly and menial occupation for a woman of her social status. She rejected a marriage proposal from a suitable gentleman and pursued her education in nursing despite her parents' disapproval.

She enrolled as a nursing student at the Lutheran Hospital of Pastor Fliedner in Kaiserwerth, Germany, in 1844. This was one of the few institutions that offered training for nurses at the time. She learned the basics of nursing care, such as hygiene, nutrition, and administration of medicines. She also observed the importance of moral and spiritual support for the patients. She admired the dedication and discipline of the deaconesses who ran the hospital.

She continued her studies at the Institute of Saint Vincent de Paul in Alexandria, Egypt, in 1850. There, she learned more about the French system of nursing, which emphasized the role of the nurse as a teacher and a leader. She also met some influential figures, such as the Sisters of Charity, who inspired her with their compassion and courage.

In 1853, she became the superintendent of the Hospital for Invalid Gentlewomen in London. She improved the conditions and standards of the hospital, and gained more experience in managing and training nurses. She also developed her skills in statistics and data analysis, which she later used to advocate for health care reform.

In 1854, she volunteered to serve as a nurse in the Crimean War, where she was put in charge of nursing British and allied soldiers in Turkey. She faced many challenges and hardships, such as lack of supplies, poor sanitation, and high mortality rates. She worked tirelessly to improve the situation, by organizing the nurses, procuring the necessary materials, and implementing strict hygiene measures. She also comforted the wounded soldiers with her personal care and attention, earning the nickname "The Lady with the Lamp".

After the war, she returned to England and established the Nightingale Training School for Nurses at St. Thomas' Hospital in London in 1860. This was the first secular nursing school in the world, and it aimed to provide a scientific and professional education for nurses. She also set up training for midwives and nurses in workhouse infirmaries. She wrote several books and reports on nursing, health, and social issues, such as Notes on Nursing (1859), Notes on Hospitals (1859), and A Contribution to the Sanitary History of the British Army (1859). She was the first woman to be awarded the Order of Merit in 1907. She died in 1910, leaving behind a legacy of nursing and health care reform.

Florence Nightingale's nursing training was a journey of discovery, challenge, and innovation. She learned from various sources and mentors, and applied her knowledge and skills to improve the health and well-being of others. She also influenced the development of nursing as a profession and a science, and inspired generations of nurses with her vision and values. She was a pioneer and a leader in the field of nursing, and a role model for women and social reformers.

- Overcoming Gender and Societal Challenges

Florence was a remarkable woman who defied the expectations and limitations imposed on her by her gender and society in the 19th century. She pursued her passion for nursing and became a pioneer and a leader in the field of healthcare, as well as a social reformer and a statistician. She faced many challenges and obstacles along the way, but she overcame them with courage, determination, and innovation. She also made significant contributions to breaking gender barriers and improving the status and opportunities for women in nursing and beyond.

The Historical Context

The 19th century was a time of rapid social, economic, and political changes in Britain and Europe. The Industrial Revolution, the French Revolution, the Napoleonic Wars, the Reform Acts, and the Crimean War were some of the major events that shaped the era. However, these changes did not benefit everyone equally, especially women. Women were largely excluded from the public sphere and confined to the domestic sphere. They had limited access to education, employment, property, and political rights. They were expected to marry, bear children, and obey their husbands. They were also subject to various legal and social restrictions, such as the Contagious Diseases Acts, which targeted women suspected of being prostitutes for compulsory examination and treatment, while ignoring the men who infected them.

Women who wanted to pursue a profession or a career faced many barriers and prejudices. Nursing was one of the few occupations that was open to women, but it was not considered a respectable or desirable one. Nursing was seen as a lowly and menial job, often performed by untrained and poorly paid women who worked in unsanitary and overcrowded hospitals. Nurses were also associated with immoral and promiscuous behavior, as they had to deal with male patients and doctors. Nursing was not a science or an art, but a service and a duty.

Florence Nightingale's Challenges and Strategies

Florence Nightingale was born into a wealthy and influential family in 1820. She had a privileged upbringing and a classical education, but she also had a strong sense of social justice and a calling to nursing from a young age. She rejected the conventional role of a woman of her class and chose to follow her ambition, despite the opposition and disapproval of her parents and society. She faced many challenges and difficulties in pursuing her nursing education and career, such as:

- Lack of formal training and recognition: Nightingale had to seek her own education and training in nursing, as there were no established institutions or standards for nursing in Britain. She enrolled as a nursing student at the Lutheran Hospital of Pastor Fliedner in Kaiserwerth, Germany, in 1844, and later at the Institute of Saint Vincent de Paul in Alexandria, Egypt, in 1850. She learned the basics of nursing care, as well as the importance of moral and spiritual support for the patients. She also met some influential figures, such as the Sisters of Charity, who inspired her with their compassion and courage. However, she did not receive any formal qualification or recognition for her studies, and she had to prove herself as a competent and professional nurse in the field.

- Resistance and hostility from the medical establishment: Nightingale faced resistance and hostility from the male-dominated medical establishment, which did not respect or value the role of nurses. She encountered this especially during the Crimean War, when she volunteered to serve as a nurse in Turkey in 1854. She was put in charge of nursing British and allied soldiers, who were suffering from wounds, infections, and diseases in filthy and overcrowded hospitals. She faced many obstacles and opposition from the army doctors and officials, who resented her authority and interference. She had to fight for the necessary supplies, equipment, and reforms to improve the conditions and standards of the hospitals. She also had to deal with the prejudice and harassment from some of the soldiers and officers, who did not appreciate her care and attention.

- Physical and mental exhaustion and illness: Nightingale worked tirelessly and selflessly to care for the sick and wounded, often at the expense of her own health and well-being. She contracted a severe infection, possibly brucellosis, during the Crimean War, which left her with chronic pain and fatigue for the rest of her life. She also suffered from depression and emotional stress, as she witnessed the horrors and sufferings of war and disease. She had to cope with the criticism and scrutiny of the public and the press, who praised her as a heroine, but also questioned her motives and methods. She had to balance her personal and professional life, as she maintained her relationships with her family and friends, as well as her colleagues and supporters.

Florence Nightingale's Contributions and Achievements

Despite the challenges and difficulties she faced, Nightingale overcame them with resilience and strategies, such as:

- Innovation and leadership: Nightingale was a visionary and a leader, who introduced new ideas and methods to nursing and healthcare. She applied her skills in statistics and data analysis, which she learned from her father, to document and demonstrate the impact of sanitation, hygiene, and nutrition on the health and mortality of the patients. She used diagrams and charts, such as the polar area diagram, to illustrate her findings and persuade the authorities and the public to support her reforms. She also developed a system of triage, which prioritized the treatment of the most urgent cases. She organized and trained the nurses, and established a hierarchy and a division of labor. She also created a rapport and a communication with the patients, and provided them with comfort and dignity.

- Education and professionalization: Nightingale was a pioneer and a founder of modern nursing, who established the first secular nursing school in the world, the Nightingale Training School for Nurses, at St. Thomas' Hospital in London in 1860. She aimed to provide a scientific and professional education for nurses, based on her own experience and knowledge. She also set up training for midwives and nurses in workhouse infirmaries, where the poor and the destitute received medical care. She wrote several books and reports on nursing, health, and social issues, such as Notes on Nursing (1859), Notes on Hospitals (1859), and A Contribution to the Sanitary

History of the British Army (1859). She also mentored and influenced many nurses and health reformers, such as Agnes Jones, Linda Richards, and Clara Barton.

- Advocacy and social reform: Nightingale was a social reformer and a humanitarian, who advocated for the improvement of the health and well-being of the people, especially the vulnerable and the marginalized. She campaigned for the repeal of the Contagious Diseases Acts, which violated the rights and dignity of women. She also supported the cause of women's suffrage, and signed the petitions for the vote for women. She also worked for the improvement of the health and sanitation of India, where she had never visited, but had a keen interest and concern. She advised the Indian government on various matters, such as irrigation, agriculture, and famine relief. She also promoted the education and employment of Indian women, especially in nursing and midwifery.

Florence Nightingale's Legacy and Impact

Florence Nightingale's journey in overcoming gender and societal challenges was a remarkable one, which left a lasting legacy and impact on nursing and healthcare, as well as on women and society. She changed the perception and the practice of nursing, from a lowly and menial occupation, to a respected and noble profession. She raised the standards and the status of nursing, and created a model and a foundation for nursing education and practice. She also improved the quality and the safety of healthcare, and reduced the suffering and the mortality of the patients. She also broke the gender barriers and the stereotypes, and opened the doors and the opportunities for women in nursing and beyond. She was a role model and an inspiration for women and social reformers, who followed her footsteps and continued her work. She was a pioneer and a leader, who made a difference in the world with her vision and her values. She was a hero and a legend, who earned the admiration and the gratitude of the people, and the recognition and the honor of the nation. She was awarded the Order of Merit in 1907, the first woman to receive this distinction. She died in 1910, at the age of 90, leaving behind a legacy of nursing and health care reform.

5. The Lady with the Lamp

- Florence's Role in the Crimean War

She played a pivotal role in the Crimean War (1853-1856), a conflict between the Russian Empire and an alliance of Britain, France, the Ottoman Empire, and Sardinia. She was in charge of nursing British and allied soldiers in Turkey, where she improved the conditions and standards of the military hospitals, reduced the mortality rates, and provided comfort and care to the wounded. She also influenced the development of nursing as a profession and a science, and advocated for health care reform and social justice.

Historical Context

The Crimean War was a result of the rivalry and tension between the Russian Empire and the Ottoman Empire over the control of the territories and the peoples in the Balkans and the Middle East. The war also involved the interests and the interventions of Britain and France, who wanted to preserve the balance of power in Europe and to protect their trade and influence in the region. The war was fought mainly in the Crimean Peninsula, where the Russians besieged the strategic port of Sevastopol, defended by the British, French, and Ottoman forces. The war also involved naval and land battles in other parts of the Black Sea, the Baltic Sea, the Caucasus, and the Danube.

The conditions of the military hospitals and the challenges faced by the medical personnel were appalling and horrific. The hospitals were overcrowded, unsanitary, and poorly supplied. The soldiers suffered from wounds, infections, diseases, and malnutrition. The medical staff were inexperienced, untrained, and overwhelmed. The army doctors and officials were resistant to change and improvement. The mortality rates were extremely high, especially from preventable causes such as cholera, typhus, and scurvy. According to some estimates, more than 16,000 British soldiers died from disease, compared to about 4,000 from battle wounds[1].

Florence's Decision and Initiatives

Florence Nightingale was the head of a nursing group in London when she heard about the plight of the British soldiers in the Crimean War. She felt a strong sense of duty and compassion to help them, and she volunteered to serve as a nurse in Turkey. She was appointed by the Secretary of War, Sidney Herbert, who was a friend and a supporter of her. She was given the authority and the resources to organize and train a team of 38 women nurses, mostly from religious orders, to accompany her to the war zone. She arrived at the British military hospital in Scutari, Turkey, in November 1854, and was shocked and appalled by what she saw. She wrote in a letter to her friend: "Hundreds of poor fellows lying on the wet ground, dying of fever, dysentery, and cholera, with no one to attend to them, no medicines, no comforts, no food but salt pork and biscuit, no clothing but their ragged uniforms, no fire, no light, no hope"[2].

She immediately set to work to improve the situation, by implementing several strategic initiatives, such as:

- Organizing and training the nurses, and establishing a hierarchy and a division of labor. She also supervised and instructed the orderlies, the soldiers, and the volunteers who assisted in the nursing care.

- Procuring and distributing the necessary supplies, equipment, and materials, such as beds, blankets, mattresses, pillows, sheets, towels, soap, basins, bandages, medicines, food, and clothing. She also solicited and received donations and contributions from the public and the press, who supported her cause and admired her work.

- Improving the sanitation and hygiene of the hospital, by cleaning and ventilating the wards, disposing of the waste and the corpses, installing proper drainage and sewerage systems, and providing clean water and fresh air. She also enforced strict rules and regulations regarding the cleanliness and the orderliness of the hospital and the staff.

- Implementing a system of triage, which prioritized the treatment of the most urgent and the most serious cases, and allocated the resources and the personnel accordingly. She also introduced a system of record-keeping and documentation, which tracked the admission, the discharge, the diagnosis, the treatment, and the outcome of the patients.

- Applying her skills in statistics and data analysis, which she learned from her father, to document and demonstrate the impact of her reforms on the health and the mortality of the patients. She used diagrams and charts, such as the polar area diagram, to illustrate her findings and persuade the authorities and the public to support her reforms. She also collected and analyzed data on various aspects of the war, such as the supply, the transport, the administration, and the logistics of the army.

- Providing comfort and care to the wounded soldiers, by attending to their physical, emotional, and spiritual needs. She also communicated and interacted with the soldiers, by listening to their stories, reading and writing letters for them, and praying with them. She earned the respect and the affection of the soldiers, who called her "The Lady with the Lamp", as she made her night rounds with a lantern in her hand.

Her Experiences and Effects

Florence Nightingale's experiences in the Crimean War were challenging and rewarding, as well as traumatic and stressful. She faced many difficulties and hardships, such as:

- Resistance and hostility from the medical establishment, which did not respect or value the role of nurses. She encountered this especially from the army doctors and officials, who resented her authority and interference. She had to fight for her reforms and prove her competence and professionalism.

- Prejudice and harassment from some of the soldiers and officers, who did not appreciate her care and attention. She had to deal with the sexism and the misogyny of the military culture, which viewed women as inferior and unwelcome.

- Physical and mental exhaustion and illness, as she worked tirelessly and selflessly to care for the sick and wounded, often at the expense of her own health and well-being. She contracted a severe infection, possibly brucellosis, during the war, which left her with chronic pain and fatigue for the rest of her life. She also suffered from depression and emotional stress, as she witnessed the horrors and sufferings of war and disease. She had to cope with the criticism and scrutiny of the public and the press, who praised her as a heroine, but also questioned her motives and methods.

- Personal and professional conflicts and dilemmas, as she had to balance her personal and professional life, and her loyalty and duty to her family, friends, colleagues, and supporters. She also had to reconcile her religious faith and her moral values with the realities and the complexities of war and politics.

She also had many achievements and successes, such as:

- Improving the conditions and standards of the military hospitals, and reducing the mortality rates of the patients. According to some estimates, she lowered the death rate from 42% to 2% in six months[3].

- Influencing the development of nursing as a profession and a science, and establishing the principles and the practices of modern nursing. She also founded the first secular nursing school in the world, the Nightingale Training School for Nurses, at St. Thomas' Hospital in London in 1860.

- Advocating for health care reform and social justice, and raising awareness and support for the improvement of the health and well-being of the people, especially the vulnerable and the marginalized. She also campaigned for the repeal of the Contagious Diseases Acts, which violated the rights and dignity of women.

- Inspiring generations of nurses and health reformers, who followed her footsteps and continued her work. She also mentored and influenced many nurses and health reformers, such as Agnes Jones, Linda Richards, and Clara Barton.

- Earning the admiration and the gratitude of the people, and the recognition and the honor of the nation. She was awarded the Order of Merit in 1907, the first woman to receive this distinction. She also received many other honors and awards, such as the Royal Red Cross, the Florence Nightingale Medal, and the Lady of Grace of the Order of St. John.

Florence Nightingale's role in the Crimean War was a significant and a remarkable one, which left a lasting impact on nursing and health care, as well as on women and society. She changed the perception and the practice of nursing, from a lowly and menial occupation, to a respected and noble profession. She raised the standards and the status of nursing, and created a model and a foundation for nursing education and practice. She also improved the quality and the safety of health care, and reduced the suffering and the mortality of the patients. She also broke the gender barriers and the stereotypes, and opened the doors and the opportunities for women in nursing and beyond. She was a role model and an inspiration for women and social reformers, who followed her footsteps and continued her work. She was a pioneer and a leader, who made a difference in the world with her vision and her values. She was a hero and a legend, who earned the admiration and the gratitude of the people, and the recognition and the honor of the nation. She died in 1910, at the age of 90, leaving behind a legacy of nursing and health care reform.

- The Iconic Image and its Symbolism

One of the most enduring and iconic images of Florence Nightingale is that of 'The Lady with the Lamp', a nickname she earned during her work at Scutari, the British military hospital in Turkey. The image depicts her as a ministering angel, walking among the beds of the sick and dying soldiers, holding a lamp in her hand. The image has a rich and nuanced symbolism, which reflects both the historical context and the lasting cultural significance of her role in the Crimean War and in the legacy of nursing.

The Historical Context

The significance of the lamp in the historical context can be understood from various perspectives, such as:

- The practical and functional perspective: The lamp was a necessary and useful tool for Nightingale and her nurses, as they worked in the dark and gloomy wards of the hospital, which lacked proper lighting and ventilation. The lamp enabled them to see and examine the patients, to administer medicines and treatments, and to perform other tasks. The lamp also helped them to navigate the corridors and the stairs of the hospital, which were often crowded and dangerous. The lamp was a symbol of their diligence and efficiency, as they worked tirelessly and selflessly to care for the sick and wounded.

- The aesthetic and artistic perspective: The lamp was a striking and beautiful contrast to the dismal and dreary surroundings of the hospital, which were filled with dirt, filth, and death. The lamp created a warm and gentle glow, which softened the harsh and grim reality of the war and the disease. The lamp also enhanced the appearance and the expression of Nightingale and her nurses, who were often dressed in simple and modest attire, and who radiated kindness and compassion. The lamp was a symbol of their grace and elegance, as they brought light and beauty to the dark and ugly world.

- The moral and spiritual perspective: The lamp was a powerful and profound metaphor for Nightingale and her nurses, as they embodied the values and the virtues of nursing and humanity. The lamp represented their wisdom and knowledge, as they applied their skills and experience to improve the health and the well-being of the patients. The lamp also represented their faith and devotion, as they followed their calling and mission to serve and heal others. The lamp was a symbol of their goodness and holiness, as they shone like stars in the night sky.

The Symbolism of the Lamp

The symbolism of the lamp in Nightingale's nighttime rounds can be explored from various angles, such as:

- The personal and individual angle: The lamp was a reflection and an expression of Nightingale's personality and character, as she demonstrated her leadership and initiative, her courage and determination, and her passion and compassion. The lamp also revealed her emotions and feelings, as she showed her sympathy and empathy, her joy and sorrow, and her love and care. The lamp was a symbol of her identity and individuality, as she distinguished herself from the others and made her mark in history.

- The social and collective angle: The lamp was a connection and a communication between Nightingale and her patients, as she established a rapport and a relationship with them, by listening to their stories, reading and writing letters for them, and praying with them. The lamp also inspired and influenced the others, such as her nurses, her colleagues, and her supporters, who admired and respected her, and who followed and assisted her. The lamp was a symbol of her role and responsibility, as she represented and advocated for the interests and the rights of the people, especially the vulnerable and the marginalized.

- The political and cultural angle: The lamp was a challenge and a critique to the status quo and the establishment, as she confronted and questioned the authority and the competence of the army and the medical officials, who opposed and resisted her reforms and innovations. The lamp also created and shaped the public opinion and the media representation, as she attracted and received the attention and the admiration of the press and the people, who supported and celebrated her cause and her work. The lamp was a symbol of her power and influence, as she changed and transformed the perception and the practice of nursing and health care, and as she broke and transcended the barriers and the stereotypes of gender and society.

The Impact of the Image

The image of 'The Lady with the Lamp' became a symbol of hope and compassion, as it captured and conveyed the essence and the significance of Nightingale's role in the

Crimean War and in the legacy of nursing. The image had a lasting and enduring impact, as it:

- Honored and commemorated Nightingale and her nurses, who sacrificed and suffered for the sake of the others, and who made a difference in the world with their vision and their values.

- Educated and informed the public and the profession, who learned and benefited from the knowledge and the experience of Nightingale and her nurses, and who adopted and applied their principles and their practices.

- Inspired and motivated the future generations of nurses and health reformers, who followed and continued the footsteps and the work of Nightingale and her nurses, and who advanced and improved the standards and the status of nursing and health care.

The image of 'The Lady with the Lamp' is one of the most iconic and enduring images of Florence Nightingale, and of nursing in general. It is a rich and nuanced symbol, which reflects both the historical context and the lasting cultural significance of her role in the Crimean War and in the legacy of nursing. It is an image that honors, educates, and inspires, and that represents hope and compassion.

6. Impact on Modern Nursing

- Reforms and Innovations

The Healthcare System during Her Time

The healthcare system during Nightingale's time was in dire need of reform, as it was characterized by:

- Lack of formal education and training for nurses: Nursing was not considered a respectable or desirable profession for women, especially for those of higher social class. Nursing was seen as a lowly and menial job, often performed by untrained and poorly paid women who worked in unsanitary and overcrowded hospitals. Nurses were also associated with immoral and promiscuous behavior, as they had to deal with male patients and doctors. Nursing was not a science or an art, but a service and a duty.

- Lack of sanitation and hygiene in hospitals: Hospitals were overcrowded, unsanitary, and poorly supplied. Patients suffered from wounds, infections, diseases, and malnutrition. Hospitals lacked proper ventilation, drainage, sewerage, and waste disposal systems. Hospitals also lacked clean water, fresh air, and adequate food and clothing for the patients. Hospitals were breeding grounds for germs and diseases, such as cholera, typhus, and scurvy, which caused high mortality rates among the patients and the staff.

- Lack of organization and administration in hospitals: Hospitals lacked a system of record-keeping and documentation, which made it difficult to track the admission, discharge, diagnosis, treatment, and outcome of the patients. Hospitals also lacked a system of triage, which prioritized the treatment of the most urgent and serious cases, and allocated the resources and personnel accordingly. Hospitals also lacked a hierarchy and a division of labor, which resulted in confusion and inefficiency among the staff.

Nightingale's Reforms and Innovations

Nightingale introduced several reforms and innovations to nursing and health care, such as:

- Establishing the first secular nursing school in the world: Nightingale founded the Nightingale Training School for

Nurses at St. Thomas' Hospital in London in 1860, with the funds she received from the public for her work in the Crimean War. She aimed to provide a scientific and professional education for nurses, based on her own experience and knowledge. She also set up training for midwives and nurses in workhouse infirmaries, where the poor and the destitute received medical care. She wrote several books and reports on nursing, health, and social issues, such as Notes on Nursing (1859), Notes on Hospitals (1859), and A Contribution to the Sanitary History of the British Army (1859). She also mentored and influenced many nurses and health reformers, such as Agnes Jones, Linda Richards, and Clara Barton.

- Improving the sanitation and hygiene of hospitals: Nightingale applied her skills in statistics and data analysis, which she learned from her father, to document and demonstrate the impact of sanitation, hygiene, and nutrition on the health and mortality of the patients. She used diagrams and charts, such as the polar area diagram, to illustrate her findings and persuade the authorities and the public to support her reforms. She also improved the conditions and standards of the hospitals, by cleaning and ventilating the wards, disposing of the waste and the corpses, installing proper drainage and sewerage systems, and providing clean water and fresh air. She also enforced strict rules and regulations regarding the cleanliness and the orderliness of the hospital and the staff.

- Implementing a system of triage, record-keeping, and administration: Nightingale introduced a system of triage, which prioritized the treatment of the most urgent and serious cases, and allocated the resources and personnel accordingly. She also introduced a system of record-keeping and documentation, which tracked the admission, discharge, diagnosis, treatment, and outcome of the patients. She also organized and trained the nurses, and established a hierarchy and a division of labor. She also created a rapport and a communication with the patients, and provided them with comfort and dignity.

- Providing comfort and care to the wounded soldiers: Nightingale communicated and interacted with the soldiers, by listening to their stories, reading and writing letters for them, and praying with them. She also attended to their physical, emotional, and spiritual needs. She earned the respect and the affection of the soldiers, who called her "The Lady with the Lamp", as she made her night rounds with a lantern in her hand.

The Challenges and the Impact of Her Initiatives

Nightingale faced many challenges and difficulties in implementing her reforms and innovations, such as:

- Resistance and hostility from the medical establishment, which did not respect or value the role of nurses. She encountered this especially during the Crimean War, when she volunteered to serve as a nurse in Turkey in 1854. She was put in charge of nursing British and allied soldiers, who were suffering from wounds, infections, and diseases in filthy and overcrowded hospitals. She faced many obstacles and opposition from the army doctors and officials, who resented her authority and interference. She had to fight for the necessary supplies, equipment, and reforms to improve the conditions and standards of the hospitals.

- Prejudice and harassment from some of the soldiers and officers, who did not appreciate her care and attention. She had to deal with the sexism and the misogyny of the military culture, which viewed women as inferior and unwelcome.

- Physical and mental exhaustion and illness, as she worked tirelessly and selflessly to care for the sick and wounded, often at the expense of her own health and well-being. She contracted a severe infection, possibly brucellosis, during the Crimean War, which left her with chronic pain and fatigue for the rest of her life. She also suffered from depression and emotional stress, as she witnessed the horrors and sufferings of war and disease. She had to cope with the criticism and scrutiny of the public and the press, who praised her as a heroine, but also questioned her motives and methods.

- Personal and professional conflicts and dilemmas, as she had to balance her personal and professional life, and her loyalty and duty to her family, friends, colleagues, and supporters. She also had to reconcile her religious faith and her moral values with the realities and the complexities of war and politics.

Nightingale's reforms and innovations had a lasting and enduring impact on nursing and health care, as they:

- Improved the quality and the safety of health care, and reduced the suffering and the mortality of the patients.

According to some estimates, she lowered the death rate from 42% to 2% in six months[3].

- Influenced the development of nursing as a profession and a science, and established the principles and the practices of modern nursing. She also founded the first secular nursing school in the world, the Nightingale Training School for Nurses, at St. Thomas' Hospital in London in 1860.

- Advocated for health care reform and social justice, and raised awareness and support for the improvement of the health and well-being of the people, especially the vulnerable and the marginalized. She also campaigned for the repeal of the Contagious Diseases Acts, which violated the rights and dignity of women.

- Inspired generations of nurses and health reformers, who followed her footsteps and continued her work. She also mentored and influenced many nurses and health reformers, such as Agnes Jones, Linda Richards, and Clara Barton.

- Earning the admiration and the gratitude of the people, and the recognition and the honor of the nation. She was awarded the Order of Merit in 1907, the first woman to receive this distinction. She also received many other honors and awards, such as the Royal Red Cross, the Florence Nightingale Medal, and the Lady of Grace of the Order of St. John.

Florence Nightingale's reforms and innovations in nursing were groundbreaking and transformative, as they changed and improved the perception and the practice of nursing and health care. She was a pioneer and a leader, who made a difference in the world with her vision and her values. She was a hero and a legend, who earned the admiration and the gratitude of the people, and the recognition and the honor of the nation. She died in 1910, at the age of 90, leaving behind a legacy of nursing and health care reform.

- Establishing Nursing as a Profession

The societal perceptions of nursing during Nightingale's time were largely negative and dismissive. Nursing was not considered a respectable or desirable profession for women, especially for those of higher social class. Nursing was seen as a lowly and menial job, often performed by untrained and poorly paid women who worked in unsanitary and overcrowded hospitals. Nurses were also associated with immoral and promiscuous behavior, as they had to deal with male patients and doctors. Nursing was not a science or an art, but a service and a duty.

Nightingale's Efforts in Elevating the Status of Nursing

Nightingale introduced several efforts and initiatives to elevate the status of nursing, such as:

- Establishing the first secular nursing school in the world: Nightingale founded the Nightingale Training School for Nurses at St. Thomas' Hospital in London in 1860, with the funds she received from the public for her work in the Crimean War. She aimed to provide a scientific and professional education for nurses, based on her own experience and knowledge. She also set up training for midwives and nurses in workhouse infirmaries, where the poor and the destitute received medical care. She wrote several books and reports on nursing, health, and social issues, such as Notes on Nursing (1859), Notes on Hospitals (1859), and A Contribution to the Sanitary History of the British Army (1859). She also mentored and influenced many nurses and health reformers, such as Agnes Jones, Linda Richards, and Clara Barton[12].

- Improving the sanitation and hygiene of hospitals: Nightingale applied her skills in statistics and data analysis, which she learned from her father, to document and demonstrate the impact of sanitation, hygiene, and nutrition on the health and mortality of the patients. She used diagrams and charts, such as the polar area diagram, to illustrate her findings and persuade the authorities and the public to support her reforms. She also improved the conditions and standards of the hospitals, by cleaning and ventilating the wards, disposing of the waste and the corpses, installing proper drainage and sewerage systems, and providing clean water and fresh air. She also enforced strict rules and regulations regarding the cleanliness and the orderliness of the hospital and the staff[34].

- Implementing a system of triage, record-keeping, and administration: Nightingale introduced a system of triage, which prioritized the treatment of the most urgent and serious cases, and allocated the resources and personnel accordingly. She also introduced a system of record-keeping and documentation, which tracked the admission, discharge, diagnosis, treatment, and outcome of the patients. She also organized and trained the nurses, and established a hierarchy and a division of labor. She also created a rapport and a communication with the patients, and provided them with comfort and dignity[5] .

- Providing comfort and care to the wounded soldiers: Nightingale communicated and interacted with the soldiers, by listening to their stories, reading and writing letters for them, and praying with them. She also attended to their physical, emotional, and spiritual needs. She earned the respect and the affection of the soldiers, who called her "The Lady with the Lamp", as she made her night rounds with a lantern in her hand .

- Advocating for health care reform and social justice: Nightingale campaigned for the improvement of the health and well-being of the people, especially the vulnerable and the marginalized. She also advocated for the repeal of the Contagious Diseases Acts, which violated the rights and dignity of women. She also supported the cause of women's suffrage, and signed the petitions for the vote for women. She also worked for the improvement of the health and sanitation of India, where she had never visited, but had a keen interest and concern. She advised the Indian government on various matters, such as irrigation, agriculture, and famine relief. She also promoted the education and employment of Indian women, especially in nursing and midwifery .

The Challenges and the Milestones of Her Initiatives

Nightingale faced many challenges and difficulties in implementing her initiatives, such as:

- Resistance and hostility from the medical establishment, which did not respect or value the role of nurses. She encountered this especially during the Crimean War, when she volunteered to serve as a nurse in Turkey in 1854. She was put in charge of nursing British and allied soldiers, who were suffering from wounds, infections, and diseases in filthy and overcrowded hospitals. She faced many obstacles and opposition from the army doctors and officials, who resented her authority and interference. She had to fight for the necessary supplies, equipment, and reforms to improve the conditions and standards of the hospitals .

- Prejudice and harassment from some of the soldiers and officers, who did not appreciate her care and attention. She had to deal with the sexism and the misogyny of the military culture, which viewed women as inferior and unwelcome .

- Physical and mental exhaustion and illness, as she worked tirelessly and selflessly to care for the sick and wounded, often at the expense of her own health and well-being. She contracted a severe infection, possibly brucellosis, during the Crimean War, which left her with chronic pain and fatigue for the rest of her life. She also suffered from depression and emotional stress, as she witnessed the horrors and sufferings of war and disease. She had to cope with the criticism and scrutiny of the public and the press, who praised her as a heroine, but also questioned her motives and methods .

- Personal and professional conflicts and dilemmas, as she had to balance her personal and professional life, and her loyalty and duty to her family, friends, colleagues, and supporters. She also had to reconcile her religious faith and her moral values with the realities and the complexities of war and politics .

Nightingale's initiatives had a lasting and enduring impact on nursing and health care, as they:

- Improved the quality and the safety of health care, and reduced the suffering and the mortality of the patients. According to some estimates, she lowered the death rate from 42% to 2% in six months[3].

- Influenced the development of nursing as a profession and a science, and established the principles and the practices of modern nursing. She also founded the first secular nursing school in the world, the Nightingale Training School for Nurses, at St. Thomas' Hospital in London in 1860.

- Advocated for health care reform and social justice, and raised awareness and support for the improvement of the health and well-being of the people, especially the vulnerable and the marginalized. She also campaigned for the repeal of the Contagious Diseases Acts, which violated the rights and dignity of women. She also supported the cause of women's suffrage, and signed the petitions for the vote for women. She also worked for the improvement of the health and sanitation of India, where she had never visited, but had a keen interest and concern. She advised the Indian government on various matters, such as irrigation, agriculture, and famine relief. She also promoted the education and employment of Indian women, especially in nursing and midwifery.

- Inspired generations of nurses and health reformers, who followed her footsteps and continued her work. She also mentored and influenced many nurses and health reformers, such as Agnes Jones, Linda Richards, and Clara Barton.

- Earning the admiration and the gratitude of the people, and the recognition and the honor of the nation. She was awarded the Order of Merit in 1907, the first woman to receive this distinction. She also received many other honors and awards, such as the Royal Red Cross, the Florence Nightingale Medal, and the Lady of Grace of the Order of St. John.

Florence Nightingale's role in establishing nursing as a profession was a significant and a remarkable one, which left a lasting impact on nursing and health care, as well as on women and society. She changed and improved the perception and the practice of nursing, from a lowly and menial occupation, to a respected and noble profession. She raised the standards and the status of nursing, and created a model and a foundation for nursing education and practice. She also improved the quality and the safety of health care, and reduced the suffering and the mortality of the patients.

She also broke the gender barriers and the stereotypes, and opened the doors and the opportunities for women in nursing and beyond. She was a pioneer and a leader, who made a difference in the world with her vision and her values. She was a hero and a legend, who earned the admiration and the gratitude of the people, and the recognition and the honor of the nation. She died in 1910, at the age of 90, leaving behind a legacy of nursing and health care reform.

7. Compassion in Action

- Stories of Florence's Compassionate Care

The healthcare environment during Nightingale's time was challenging and emotionally draining. The hospitals were overcrowded, unsanitary, and poorly supplied. The soldiers suffered from wounds, infections, diseases, and malnutrition. The medical staff were inexperienced, untrained, and overwhelmed. The army doctors and officials were resistant to change and improvement. The mortality rates were extremely high, especially from preventable causes such as cholera, typhus, and scurvy. According to some estimates, more than 16,000 British soldiers died from disease, compared to about 4,000 from battle wounds[1].

Nightingale demonstrated exceptional compassion in her care of the patients, as she:

- Volunteered to serve as a nurse in Turkey, despite the opposition and hostility of her family, friends, and the medical establishment. She felt a strong sense of duty and compassion to help the soldiers, and she risked her own health and safety to do so. She wrote in a letter to her friend: "I am well and happy, and never was so before, because I never did what I thought right before. I have no misgivings, no doubts, no fears, no regrets"[2].

- Organized and trained a team of 38 women nurses, mostly from religious orders, to accompany her to the war zone. She was appointed by the Secretary of War, Sidney Herbert, who was a friend and a supporter of her. She was given the authority and the resources to organize and improve the nursing care in the military hospitals. She arrived at the British military hospital in Scutari, Turkey, in November 1854, and was shocked and appalled by what she saw. She wrote in a letter to her friend: "Hundreds of poor fellows lying on the wet ground, dying of fever, dysentery, and cholera, with no one to attend to them, no medicines, no comforts, no food but salt pork and biscuit, no clothing but their ragged uniforms, no fire, no light, no hope"[2].

- Implemented several reforms and innovations to improve the sanitation, hygiene, and nutrition of the hospital, by cleaning and ventilating the wards, disposing of the waste and the corpses, installing proper drainage and sewerage systems, and providing clean water and fresh air. She also procured and distributed the necessary supplies, equipment, and materials, such as beds, blankets, mattresses, pillows, sheets, towels, soap, basins, bandages, medicines, food, and clothing. She also solicited and received donations and contributions from the public and the press, who supported her cause and admired her work.

- Applied her skills in statistics and data analysis, which she learned from her father, to document and demonstrate the impact of her reforms on the health and the mortality of the patients. She used diagrams and charts, such as the polar area diagram, to illustrate her findings and persuade the authorities and the public to support her reforms. She also collected and analyzed data on various aspects of the war, such as the supply, the transport, the administration, and the logistics of the army.

- Implemented a system of triage, which prioritized the treatment of the most urgent and the most serious cases, and allocated the resources and the personnel accordingly. She also introduced a system of record-keeping and documentation, which tracked the admission, the discharge, the diagnosis, the treatment, and the outcome of the patients. She also organized and trained the nurses, and established a hierarchy and a division of labor. She also supervised and instructed the orderlies, the soldiers, and the volunteers who assisted in the nursing care.

- Provided comfort and care to the wounded soldiers, by attending to their physical, emotional, and spiritual needs. She also communicated and interacted with the soldiers, by listening to their stories, reading and writing letters for them, and praying with them. She earned the respect and the affection of the soldiers, who called her "The Lady with the Lamp", as she made her night rounds with a lantern in her hand.

Nightingale's interactions with the patients were marked by human connection and empathy, as she:

- Treated the patients with dignity and respect, regardless of their rank, nationality, religion, or background. She cared for the British, French, Turkish, and Russian soldiers alike, and even for the animals that accompanied them. She wrote in a letter to her friend: "I never made the distinction between Turk and Christian, between English and French, between man and beast. I have nursed them all alike"[2].

- Showed kindness and compassion to the patients, by providing them with not only medical care, but also personal care. She washed and groomed them, changed their dressings and linens, fed and hydrated them, and comforted and consoled them. She wrote in a letter to her friend: "I have never seen such suffering as I have here. I have never seen such wounds as I have here. I have never seen such courage as I have here. I have never seen such gratitude as I have here"[2].

- Established a rapport and a relationship with the patients, by learning their names, their stories, their families, and their preferences. She also helped them to keep in touch with their loved ones, by reading and writing letters for them, and sending them gifts and tokens. She wrote in a letter to her friend: "I know every man's face, every man's name, every man's history, every man's hopes and fears. I am their mother, their sister, their friend"[2].

- Inspired and influenced the patients, by giving them hope, courage, and faith. She also encouraged them to participate in their own recovery, by engaging them in activities, such as games, music, and crafts. She wrote in a letter to her friend: "I have seen men who were dying of despair, who were revived by a word, a smile, a touch. I have seen men who were dying of pain, who were relieved by a song, a prayer, a flower. I have seen men who were dying of disease, who were cured by a medicine, a surgery, a miracle".

- Humanitarian Efforts Beyond the Battlefield

Florence is undoubtedly most recognized for her revolutionary work in battlefield nursing during the Crimean War. However, her unwavering dedication to public health and social reform extended far beyond the trenches, leaving an indelible mark on 19th-century society and influencing public health policies to this day.

Victorian England, the backdrop for Nightingale's endeavors, was riddled with societal challenges and health issues. Poor sanitation, overcrowding, and rampant poverty fueled epidemics like cholera and typhus, disproportionately impacting the working class. These realities ignited a deep-seated compassion in Nightingale, urging her to advocate for a holistic approach to healthcare that transcended mere bedside care.

Her initiatives reached beyond the traditional healthcare settings of hospitals. Through statistical analysis, she meticulously gathered data on sanitation and hygiene practices, exposing the link between unsanitary conditions and high death rates. This groundbreaking work led to her influential "Notes on Nursing," an early handbook promoting evidence-based hygiene practices within hospitals and homes.

Nightingale became a relentless advocate for social reforms. She lobbied for improved sanitation infrastructure, affordable housing, and better nutrition programs for the underprivileged. Her relentless campaigning for public health measures like regular waste collection and clean water provision demonstrably reduced disease outbreaks, demonstrating the undeniable societal benefits of preventive healthcare.

Furthermore, she recognized the crucial role of education in empowering individuals to contribute to their own well-being. She established the Nightingale Training School, which instilled in nurses not just clinical skills but also a dedication to community health education. This focus on empowering individuals resonated throughout her initiatives, from promoting female healthcare education to advocating for improved health awareness campaigns targeting the general public.

The impact of Nightingale's humanitarian endeavors on broader societal well-being is undeniable. Her tireless efforts resulted in significant improvements in public health infrastructure, leading to a decline in preventable diseases and a rise in life expectancy across all social classes. Her advocacy for social reforms paved the way for improved living conditions, particularly for the working class and marginalized communities.

Most importantly, Florence Nightingale's legacy lies in her holistic approach to healthcare. She understood that health is not merely the absence of disease but rather a complex interplay of social, environmental, and individual factors. This groundbreaking perspective revolutionized the field of public health, shifting the focus towards prevention, education, and empowering communities to actively participate in their own well-being.

Her unwavering commitment to public health and social reform continues to inspire and shape policies even today. From global sanitation initiatives to community-based health education programs, her legacy echoes in countless efforts to create a healthier and more equitable world. Florence Nightingale's vision remains a vital reminder that true public health requires not just doctors and nurses, but a collective effort to address the social and environmental determinants of well-being, ensuring a healthier future for generations to come.

8. Personal Life

Florence Nightingale was a remarkable woman who defied the conventional expectations of her time and pursued her passion for nursing and social reform. Her personal life was shaped by her spiritual convictions, her intellectual curiosity, and her strong sense of duty.

In the 19th century, women were expected to remain subservient to their fathers and husbands, and their occupational choices were extremely limited[1]. Middle- and upper-class women generally remained home, caring for their children and running the household[1]. They were not allowed to be outspoken, and they were not given the same opportunities as men[3]. Nightingale, however, rejected these norms and chose a different path for herself.

Nightingale felt a calling to serve God and humanity through nursing since she was a young girl[4]. She believed that nursing was her divine purpose and that she had a moral obligation to fulfill it[5]. She faced opposition from her parents, who forbade her to pursue nursing and wanted her to marry a wealthy man[45]. Nightingale refused several marriage proposals, including one from Richard Monckton Milnes, a politician and poet who courted her for nine years[47]. She explained her reason for turning him down, saying that while he stimulated her intellectually and romantically, her "moral…active nature…requires satisfaction, and that would not find it in this life"[5].

Nightingale was determined to pursue her true calling despite her parents' objections, and she sought education and training in nursing at various institutions, such as the Lutheran Hospital of Pastor Fliedner in Kaiserwerth, Germany[45]. She also traveled extensively and learned from different cultures and health systems[45]. She gained knowledge and experience that prepared her for her future leadership roles in nursing and public health.

Nightingale's professional life was marked by many achievements and challenges. She rose to fame for her work during the Crimean War, where she improved the sanitary conditions and reduced the mortality rates of wounded soldiers[45]. She spent many hours in the wards, and her night rounds giving personal care to the wounded established her image as the "Lady with the Lamp"[45]. Her efforts to formalize nursing education led her to establish the first scientifically based nursing school—the Nightingale School of Nursing, at St. Thomas' Hospital in London (opened 1860)[45]. She also was instrumental in setting up training for midwives and nurses in workhouse infirmaries[45]. She also advocated for various causes, such as sanitary and social reforms, public health policies, hunger relief, women's education, and human rights[456].

Nightingale's professional life, however, also took a toll on her personal life. She suffered from chronic illnesses, such as brucellosis, depression, and post-traumatic stress disorder[45]. She also faced criticism and resistance from some of her colleagues, superiors, and politicians, who did not appreciate her innovations and reforms.

Nightingale's personal life was also enriched by her relationships and friendships with various people, who supported her, inspired her, and challenged her. She had a close bond with her sister, Parthenope, who was her companion and confidante[45]. She also had several important and passionate friendships with women, such as Mary

Clarke, an Englishwoman she met in 1837 and kept in touch with throughout her life[68]. She also corresponded with Irish nun Sister Mary Clare Moore, with whom she had worked in Crimea[6]. She also had influential mentors and allies, such as Sidney Herbert, the secretary of war who appointed her to lead the nursing team in Crimea[45], and Benjamin Jowett, the master of Balliol College, Oxford, who encouraged her to write and publish her works[45]. She also had numerous godchildren, whom she loved and cared for.

Nightingale's personal life was a complex and fascinating one, that revealed the woman behind the pioneering nurse. She was a visionary, a leader, a reformer, and a humanitarian, who devoted her life to improving the health and well-being of others. She was also a human being, who had her own struggles, doubts, fears, and joys. She was a woman who balanced her personal and professional obligations, and who followed her own path, despite the challenges and obstacles she faced. She was a woman who made a difference in the world, and who continues to inspire generations of nurses and health care professionals.

9. Marriage and Family

- Florence's Relationship and Marriage

In the 19th century, marriage was considered the natural and desirable state for women, especially for those of the upper and middle classes. Women were expected to marry young, bear children, and devote themselves to their husbands and families. They were not supposed to pursue careers or public roles, and they were denied the same rights and opportunities as men. Marriage was also a matter of social and economic status, and women were often pressured to marry men of wealth and influence, regardless of their personal preferences[12].

Nightingale, however, rejected these norms and chose a different path for herself. She felt a calling to serve God and humanity through nursing since she was a young girl[3]. She believed that nursing was her divine purpose and that she had a moral obligation to fulfill it[4]. She faced opposition from her parents, who forbade her to pursue nursing and wanted her to marry a wealthy man[34].

Nightingale refused several marriage proposals, including one from Richard Monckton Milnes, a politician and poet who courted her for nine years[3] . She explained her reason for turning him down, saying that while he stimulated her intellectually and romantically, her "moral...active nature...requires satisfaction, and that would not find it in this life"[4].

Nightingale never married and had no children. Her work was her legacy. She devoted her life to improving the health and well-being of others, especially the wounded soldiers, the poor, and the oppressed. She was a pioneer and a leader in nursing and public health, and she influenced the quality of care and the professionalization of nursing in the 19th and 20th centuries[34] .

Nightingale's decision to remain single and pursue her career was not an easy one. She faced many challenges and sacrifices, both personally and professionally. She suffered from chronic illnesses, such as brucellosis, depression, and post-traumatic stress disorder, which affected her physical and mental health[34]. She also faced criticism and resistance from some of her colleagues, superiors, and politicians, who did not appreciate her innovations and reforms[34]. She also struggled with the ethical dilemmas and moral conflicts that arose from her involvement in war and colonialism.

- Family Dynamics and Support

Florence Nightingale's family life was a complex and influential factor in her personal and professional development. She was born into a wealthy and prominent British family, who had high expectations and social ambitions for their children. However, she also had a strong sense of individuality and a calling to serve God and humanity through nursing, which often clashed with her family's wishes and norms.

In the 19th century, the family was considered the basic unit of society and the main source of identity and support for individuals. The family was also a site of socialization, where children learned the values, norms, and roles of their culture and class. The family was also a site of conflict, where power and authority were exercised and challenged, and where personal and collective interests were negotiated and balanced.

Nightingale's relationship with her family was marked by both love and tension. She had a close bond with her sister, Parthenope, who was her companion and confidante. They shared many interests and experiences, such as traveling, reading, and writing. Parthenope was also supportive of Nightingale's nursing career, and helped her with administrative and financial matters.

Nightingale's relationship with her parents was more complicated. Her father, William, was a wealthy landowner and a liberal thinker, who provided her with a classical education and encouraged her intellectual pursuits. He also respected her independence and allowed her to travel and study nursing, despite his initial reluctance. He was proud of her achievements and defended her against critics.

Her mother, Frances, was a socialite and a conservative, who wanted her daughters to marry well and conform to the expectations of their class and gender. She disapproved of Nightingale's nursing career and tried to persuade her to give it up. She was also jealous of her fame and influence, and felt neglected by her. She often complained and criticized Nightingale, and made her feel guilty and ungrateful.

Nightingale's family life was also affected by her chronic illnesses, which began after her return from the Crimean War. She suffered from brucellosis, depression, and post-traumatic stress disorder, which made her physically weak and emotionally unstable. She spent most of her time in bed, and relied on her family and friends for care and comfort. She also communicated with them through letters and visits, and kept them informed of her work and ideas.

Nightingale's family life was a source of both support and challenge for her. Her family provided her with the material and emotional resources that enabled her to pursue her education and career. They also recognized and appreciated her contributions to nursing and public health, and celebrated her achievements and honors. However, her family also imposed constraints and pressures on her, and sometimes opposed and criticized her choices and actions.

They also demanded her attention and affection, and sometimes made her feel guilty and unhappy.

Nightingale's family life was a dynamic and influential factor in her personal and professional development. She was shaped by her family's values, norms, and roles, but she also challenged and changed them. She was supported by her family's love, but she also struggled with their expectations. She was a daughter, a sister, a godmother, and a friend, but she was also a nurse, a leader, a reformer, and a humanitarian. She was a woman who balanced her personal and professional obligations, and who followed her own path, despite the challenges and obstacles she faced. She was a woman who made a difference in the world, and who continues to inspire generations of nurses and health care professionals.

10. Legacy and Recognition

- *Posthumous Honors and Acknowledgments With Her Enduring Influence*

After her death in 1910, Nightingale's legacy was honored and acknowledged in various ways, both nationally and internationally. Some of the honors and acknowledgments she received posthumously were:

- The Florence Nightingale Medal, established by the International Committee of the Red Cross in 1912, which is awarded every two years to nurses or nursing aides who have shown exceptional courage and devotion to the wounded, sick, or disabled, or to civilian victims of a conflict or disaster[1].

- The Florence Nightingale Declaration, adopted by the Nightingale Initiative for Global Health in 2008, which is a global campaign to strengthen nursing and midwifery, and to advance health for all[2].

- The Florence Nightingale Museum, opened in 1989 at St. Thomas' Hospital in London, which displays her personal belongings, letters, books, and artifacts, and tells the story of her life and achievements[3].

- The Florence Nightingale Foundation, established in 1929, which provides scholarships, research grants, and leadership programs for nurses and midwives in the United Kingdom[4].

- The Florence Nightingale Faculty of Nursing, Midwifery & Palliative Care, established in 2014 at King's College London, which is the successor of the original Nightingale Training School for Nurses, and is one of the leading nursing schools in the world.

Nightingale's legacy also continues to influence modern healthcare and nursing practices, as her ideas and principles remain relevant and applicable today. Some of the enduring influences of Nightingale are:

- Her emphasis on evidence-based practice and data-driven decision making, which she demonstrated through her use of statistics, graphs, and reports to support her arguments and proposals for health reforms.

- Her holistic approach to health and well-being, which she advocated through her recognition of the multiple factors that affect health, such as environmental, social, economic, and political conditions, and her promotion of preventive measures and interventions.

- Her vision of nursing as a profession and a science, which she advanced through her establishment of the first secular nursing school, her development of a curriculum and standards for nursing education and training, and her publication of various works on nursing theory and practice.

- Her role as an advocate and a leader, which she exemplified through her tireless efforts to improve the health and welfare of various populations, such as the wounded soldiers, the poor, the oppressed, and the women, and her influence on the development of nursing and health care in various countries and regions.

Florence Nightingale's legacy and recognition are testament to her remarkable achievements and contributions to nursing and public health. She was a pioneer and a leader, a reformer and a humanitarian, who devoted her life to improving the health and well-being of others. She was a woman who made a difference in the world, and who continues to inspire generations of nurses and health care professionals..

11. Adventures Beyond Nursing

- Florence's Exploration, Travels and Pursuits Outside of the Nursing Field

Nightingale was an avid traveler, who visited various countries and regions in Europe, Asia, and Africa. She traveled with her family, friends, or companions, and sometimes alone. She traveled for different purposes, such as education, exploration, or service. Some of the places she traveled to and the reasons behind her travels were:

- Germany: She enrolled as a nursing student at the Lutheran Hospital of Pastor Fliedner in Kaiserwerth, where she received her first formal training in nursing.

- Egypt: She visited the ancient monuments and temples, and studied the history and culture of the country. She also met Gustave Flaubert, a French novelist, and Samuel Carter Hall, an Irish journalist.

- Greece: She admired the classical art and architecture, and learned about the Greek mythology and philosophy. She also witnessed the aftermath of the Greek War of Independence, and sympathized with the Greek cause.

- Turkey: She was appointed by Sidney Herbert, the secretary of war, to lead a team of nurses to care for the wounded soldiers during the Crimean War. She improved the sanitary conditions and reduced the mortality rates of the soldiers. She also collected data and wrote reports on the health situation and the medical administration of the war[45].

- France: She visited Paris and met with various political and intellectual figures, such as Alexis de Tocqueville, a French historian and politician, and Jean Henri Dunant, a Swiss humanitarian and the founder of the Red Cross.

- Italy: She explored the art and culture of the country, and met with Florence Nightingale Shaw, a distant cousin and a fellow nurse, who named her daughter after Nightingale[4].

- India: She never visited India herself, but she served as an authority on public sanitation issues in India for both the military and civilians. She wrote a report on the health of the Indian army, and proposed sanitary and social reforms for the country.

Nightingale was also a prolific and influential writer, who wrote on various topics, such as nursing, health, statistics, religion, philosophy, and social reform. She published several books and reports, such as Notes on Nursing, Notes on Hospitals, A Contribution to the Sanitary History of the British Army, and Suggestions for Thought. She also wrote hundreds of letters and articles, which she sent to her family, friends, colleagues, and authorities. She used her writing skills to communicate her ideas and proposals, to educate and inform the public, and to advocate and campaign for her causes.

Nightingale's adventures beyond nursing revealed her as a multifaceted individual, who had a wide range of interests and talents. She was a curious and adventurous traveler, a prolific and influential writer, and a passionate and visionary reformer. She was a woman who balanced her personal and professional obligations, and who followed her own path, despite the challenges and obstacles she faced. She was a woman who made a difference in the world, and who continues to inspire generations of nurses and health care professionals.

12. Pioneering Spirit

- Florence's Leadership and Vision

Nightingale's leadership style was marked by her ability to inspire and motivate others. She was able to rally support for her reforms and persuade others to adopt her ideas, even when they faced resistance. She was also known for her ability to work effectively with a wide range of people, including doctors, nurses, and hospital administrators. She was not afraid to challenge the status quo and advocate for change, using evidence and data to support her arguments. She was also a visionary who saw the big picture and the long-term goals, while being attentive to the details and the immediate needs.

Nightingale's vision for nursing and healthcare was based on the principles of prevention, holistic care, and evidence-based practice. She believed that nursing was a distinct profession from medicine, with its own body of knowledge and skills. She emphasized the importance of creating a healthy environment for the patients, addressing not only their physical needs, but also their psychological, social, and spiritual needs. She also advocated for the education and training of nurses, as well as the collection and analysis of data to improve the quality and outcomes of care. She wrote several books and reports on nursing, hospitals, and public health, which influenced the development of nursing theory, education, and practice around the world.

Nightingale's legacy is still relevant and influential today, as nurses continue to face the challenges and opportunities of providing care in a complex and changing healthcare system. Nightingale's vision for nursing as a profession that promotes health, prevents disease, and cares for the whole person is still the core of nursing practice. Her contribution to nursing research, education, and leadership is still recognized and valued. Her example of courage, compassion, and commitment is still an inspiration for nurses and other healthcare professionals. Nightingale was a trailblazer in the field of nursing, and her impact is still felt today.

- *Advocacy for Healthcare Reforms*

As you already know, one of the main healthcare challenges that Nightingale encountered during her time was the lack of sanitation and hygiene in hospitals and other settings. She witnessed the devastating effects of infections, diseases, and mortality among the soldiers and civilians during the Crimean War, where she served as a nurse and a manager. She realized that many of the deaths could have been prevented by improving the environmental conditions, such as ventilation, cleanliness, drainage, and nutrition. She collected and analyzed data to demonstrate the correlation between sanitation and health outcomes, and published her findings in reports and diagrams that were widely circulated and influential. She also implemented practical measures to improve the sanitation and hygiene in the hospitals, such as scrubbing the floors, washing the linens, disposing of the waste, and providing fresh food and water.

Another healthcare challenge that Nightingale faced was the lack of professional standards and education for nurses. She observed that many of the nurses who worked in the hospitals and the workhouses were untrained, unskilled, and undisciplined. She believed that nursing was a noble and important profession that required a solid foundation of knowledge, skills, and ethics. She established the Nightingale School of Nursing at St. Thomas' Hospital in London in 1860, which was the first secular and modern nursing school in the world. She designed the curriculum and the training program for the nurses, which included both theoretical and practical components, as well as moral and spiritual guidance. She also mentored and supported the graduates of her school, who became known as the Nightingale nurses, and encouraged them to spread her nursing principles and practices around the world.

A third healthcare challenge that Nightingale tackled was the need for healthcare reforms in the public sector, especially in the workhouses and in India. She advocated for the improvement of the health and welfare of the poor and the marginalized, who often suffered from neglect, abuse, and exploitation in the workhouses and the colonies. She proposed a reform of the workhouse infirmaries to make them high-quality taxpayer-funded hospitals, and also worked on sanitary and social reforms in India[34]. She used her political connections and her persuasive skills to lobby for her reforms, and wrote numerous letters, articles, and books to raise awareness and generate support for her causes. She also collaborated with other reformers and experts, such as Edwin Chadwick, Henry Bonham Carter, and John Sutherland, to advance her causes.

Nightingale's advocacy for healthcare reforms was not without challenges and opposition. She faced resistance from some of the medical authorities, who were skeptical of her methods and motives, and from some of the political and social elites, who were reluctant to change the status quo. She also faced personal challenges, such as her chronic illness, her family conflicts, and her isolation. She overcame these challenges by relying on her faith, her passion, and her determination. She also leveraged her reputation, her network, and her evidence to persuade and influence others.

Nightingale's advocacy for healthcare reforms had a profound and lasting impact on the healthcare system and the society. She improved the health and survival of countless patients and populations, by reducing the rates of infections, diseases, and mortality. She elevated the status and the standards of nursing as a profession, by establishing the first nursing school and the first nursing code of ethics. She also contributed to the development of healthcare policies and practices, by influencing the legislation, the administration, and the public opinion on various healthcare issues. She was widely recognized and respected as a leader and a reformer, and received many honors and awards for her work. She was also an inspiration and a role model for many nurses and other healthcare professionals, who followed her footsteps and continued her legacy. Nightingale was a trailblazer in the field of healthcare, and her impact is still felt today.

13. Lessons for Kids

- Inspirational Takeaways for Young Readers

From what you have Read, Do you know who Florence Nightingale was?

She was a famous nurse who changed the world with her courage, kindness, and intelligence. She was also a leader, a reformer, and a visionary who had a big dream of making the world a better place. Her life story is full of challenges, adventures, and achievements that can inspire and motivate you to follow your own dreams and passions.

Here are some of the lessons and values that you can learn from Florence Nightingale's life:

- Perseverance: Florence Nightingale never gave up on her goals, even when she faced difficulties and obstacles. She worked hard and persisted in pursuing her calling to nursing, despite the opposition of her family and the society. She also overcame her own illness, isolation, and exhaustion to continue her work and her reforms. She showed that perseverance is the key to success and happiness.

- Compassion: Florence Nightingale cared deeply for the people who were suffering and in need of help. She treated the patients with respect and dignity, and provided them with comfort and relief. She also advocated for the rights and welfare of the poor and the marginalized, and worked to improve their health and living conditions. She showed that compassion is the essence of nursing and humanity.

- The pursuit of one's passions: Florence Nightingale followed her heart and her passions, and did what she loved and believed in. She was passionate about nursing, statistics, and public health, and used her talents and skills to make a difference in these fields. She also enjoyed learning, writing, and traveling, and explored various topics and places. She showed that the pursuit of one's passions is the source of fulfillment and joy.

You can apply these takeaways in your own life by:

- Setting goals and working towards them: You can think about what you want to achieve in your life, and make a plan to reach your goals. You can also break down your goals into smaller and manageable steps, and track your progress and achievements. You can also seek feedback and support from others, and learn from your mistakes and failures. You can also celebrate your successes and reward yourself for your efforts.

- Being kind and helpful to others: You can show empathy and understanding to the people around you, and try to see things from their perspective. You can also offer your help and support to those who are in need, and volunteer for a good cause. You can also express your gratitude and appreciation to the people who help and inspire you, and spread positivity and happiness to others.

- Discovering and pursuing your interests and hobbies: You can explore different subjects and activities that interest you, and find out what you are good at and enjoy doing. You can also join clubs, groups, or classes that match your interests and hobbies, and meet new friends who share your passions. You can also challenge yourself to learn new skills and knowledge, and expand your horizons.

Florence Nightingale's life is an example of how one person can make a big impact on the world with their passion, compassion, and perseverance. You can also be like her, and follow your dreams and passions, and make the world a better place. Remember, you have the power and the potential to do great things, and you are never too young to start. Be inspired by Florence Nightingale, and be an inspiration to others.

- Applying Florence's Values in Today's World

Her principles of compassion, innovation, and advocacy are still relevant and needed in today's world, where many societal and healthcare issues pose challenges to the health and well-being of people and communities.

Some of the current societal and healthcare issues that affect the world today are:

- Financial difficulties: Many health systems are facing financial difficulties due to the COVID-19 pandemic, staffing problems, reduced patient volumes, and rising inflation[1]. These difficulties can compromise the quality and safety of care, and increase the health disparities among different populations.

- Health system mergers: The trend of health system mergers is expected to continue as health systems seek to expand their market share, reduce their costs, and increase their bargaining power with insurers[1]. However, mergers can also have negative impacts on the access, affordability, and diversity of care, and create conflicts of interest and ethical dilemmas for health professionals.

- Recruiting and retaining staff: The shortage of health workers is a global problem that affects the delivery and outcomes of care[2]. The COVID-19 pandemic has exacerbated the situation, as many health workers have experienced burnout, stress, and trauma. The lack of professional standards and education, the low wages and benefits, and the unsafe and unsupportive work environments are some of the factors that contribute to the recruitment and retention challenges.

- Health inequities: Health inequities are the unfair and avoidable differences in health status and outcomes among different groups of people, based on their social, economic, or environmental conditions[3]. Some of the social factors that influence health inequities are class, income, legal status, race, ethnicity, gender, sexuality, disability, and region[2]. Health inequities can lead to increased morbidity and mortality, reduced quality of life, and increased health care costs.

- Infectious diseases: Infectious diseases are caused by microorganisms, such as bacteria, viruses, fungi, and parasites, that can spread from person to person, or from animals to humans[4]. Some of the infectious diseases that pose a threat to global health are COVID-19, HIV/AIDS, tuberculosis, malaria, hepatitis, and neglected tropical diseases. Infectious diseases can cause significant morbidity and mortality, especially among vulnerable and marginalized populations, and can also have social, economic, and environmental impacts.

- Noncommunicable diseases: Noncommunicable diseases are chronic diseases that are not caused by infectious agents, but by genetic, physiological, environmental, or behavioral factors[4]. Some of the common noncommunicable diseases are cardiovascular diseases, cancer, diabetes, chronic respiratory diseases, and mental disorders. Noncommunicable diseases are the leading cause of death and disability worldwide, and are associated with risk factors such as tobacco use, unhealthy diet, physical inactivity, and harmful use of alcohol.

These are some of the examples of the complex and interrelated challenges that affect the health of individuals and communities in the 21st century. To address these challenges, we can learn from and apply the values of Florence Nightingale, who was a leader and a reformer in the field of healthcare. Some of the values that she upheld and demonstrated in her work are:

- Compassion: Compassion is the feeling of empathy and sympathy for the suffering of others, and the desire to alleviate their pain and distress. Nightingale showed compassion for the patients and the populations that she served, by providing them with holistic and humane care, and by advocating for their rights and welfare. Compassion is essential for health professionals, as it can improve the quality of care, the patient satisfaction, and the health outcomes. Compassion can also benefit the health professionals themselves, as it can reduce their stress, enhance their well-being, and increase their resilience.

- Innovation: Innovation is the process of creating or improving something new, useful, or valuable. Nightingale was an innovator who used her knowledge, skills, and creativity to transform the healthcare system. She introduced new methods and practices, such as sanitation, statistics, and education, to improve the health and survival of the patients and the public. Innovation is vital for health professionals, as it can help them to solve problems, adapt to changes, and achieve goals. Innovation can also foster the development of new technologies, services, and policies that can enhance the health of individuals and communities.

- Advocacy: Advocacy is the act of speaking or acting on behalf of oneself or others, especially those who are vulnerable or marginalized, to promote or protect their interests, rights, or needs. Nightingale was an advocate who used her influence and evidence to lobby for healthcare reforms, such as the improvement of hospital conditions, the professionalization of nursing, and the public health interventions. Advocacy is important for health professionals, as it can help them to raise awareness, mobilize resources, and influence decisions that affect the health of individuals and communities. Advocacy can also empower the health professionals and the people they serve, by giving them a voice and a choice in their health and well-being.

These are some of the values that Florence Nightingale embodied and exemplified in her life and work, and that we can emulate and apply in our own contexts. Some of the actionable steps that we can take to embody these values are:

- Practice compassion: We can practice compassion by being attentive and responsive to the needs and feelings of ourselves and others, and by providing comfort and support. We can also practice compassion by being respectful and inclusive of the diversity and dignity of ourselves and others, and by avoiding judgment and discrimination. We can also practice compassion by being grateful and appreciative of ourselves and others, and by expressing kindness and generosity.

- Foster innovation: We can foster innovation by being curious and open-minded about new ideas and opportunities, and by seeking and sharing knowledge and information. We can also foster innovation by being creative and resourceful in finding and implementing solutions, and by experimenting and learning from failures. We can also foster innovation by being collaborative and cooperative with others, and by building and participating in networks and communities of practice.

- Engage in advocacy: We can engage in advocacy by being informed and aware of the issues and challenges that affect the health of ourselves and others, and by collecting and analyzing data and evidence. We can also engage in advocacy by being proactive and assertive in expressing and defending our opinions and positions, and by communicating and negotiating with others. We can also engage in advocacy by being active and involved in the health-related activities and initiatives, and by supporting and joining the movements and organizations that work for health.

By following these steps, we can embody the values of Florence Nightingale, and contribute to the improvement of the health and well-being of ourselves and others. We can also honor the legacy of Florence Nightingale, and celebrate the Year of the Nurse and the Midwife, by recognizing and appreciating the vital role that nurses and midwives play in providing health services around the world. Florence Nightingale's values, vision, and voice are still relevant and needed in today's world, and we can learn from and apply them to address the modern-day challenges.

14. Fun Facts and Activities

- *Engaging Trivia and Quizzes*

Trivia

- Florence Nightingale was born in Florence, Italy, on May 12, 1820. She was named after the city of her birth. Her parents were wealthy and well-traveled English people, who had two daughters: Florence and her older sister, Parthenope.

- Florence Nightingale felt a strong calling to nursing from a young age. She believed that God had a special purpose for her life, and that she had to serve others, especially the poor and the sick. She wrote in her diary: "God spoke to me and called me to His service." However, her family and the society of her time did not approve of her choice, as nursing was considered a lowly and unsuitable occupation for a woman of her class and education.

- Florence Nightingale became famous during the Crimean War (1853-1856), when she led a team of nurses to care for the British soldiers who were wounded and dying in the military hospitals in Turkey. She improved the conditions and the outcomes of the hospitals by introducing sanitation, ventilation, nutrition, and organization. She also gained the respect and admiration of the soldiers and the public, who nicknamed her "the Lady with the Lamp" for her nightly rounds to comfort the patients.

- Florence Nightingale was also a pioneer of statistics and data visualization. She collected and analyzed data on the health and mortality of the soldiers and the civilians, and used them to support her arguments and proposals for healthcare reforms. She also invented a type of pie chart called the polar area diagram or the Nightingale rose diagram, which she used to illustrate the causes of death in the hospitals.

- Florence Nightingale established the first secular and modern nursing school in the world, the Nightingale School of Nursing at St. Thomas' Hospital in London, in 1860. She designed the curriculum and the training program for the nurses, which included both theoretical and practical components, as well as moral and spiritual guidance. She also mentored and supported the graduates of her school, who became known as the Nightingale nurses, and encouraged them to spread her nursing principles and practices around the world.

- Florence Nightingale suffered from a chronic illness that affected her health and mobility for most of her life. She contracted brucellosis, a bacterial infection, during the Crimean War, which caused her severe pain, fatigue, and depression. She spent much of her time in bed or on a couch, and rarely left her home. She continued her work and her reforms through writing and correspondence, and used her reputation and influence to lobby for her causes.

- Florence Nightingale received many honors and awards for her work and her reforms, such as the Order of Merit, the Royal Red Cross, and the Lady of Grace of the Order of St. John. She also became the first woman to be awarded the Freedom of the City of London and the first woman to be a member of the Royal Statistical Society. She also received honorary degrees from several universities, such as Harvard, Yale, and Oxford.

- Florence Nightingale died on August 13, 1910, at the age of 90, in her home in London. She was buried in a simple grave in the family plot in Hampshire, England, according to her wishes. She left behind a legacy of nursing theory, education, and practice, as well as healthcare policies and practices, that influenced the development of nursing and healthcare around the world. She was also an inspiration and a role model for many nurses and other healthcare professionals, who followed her footsteps and continued her legacy.

Quizzes

- What was the name of Florence Nightingale's older sister?

    - A) Frances

    - B) Parthenope

    - C) Penelope

    - D) Philippa

    - Answer: B) Parthenope

- What was the nickname given to Florence Nightingale by the soldiers and the public during the Crimean War?

    - A) The Lady with the Lamp

    - B) The Angel of Mercy

    - C) The Queen of Nurses

    - D) The Mother of Medicine

    - Answer: A) The Lady with the Lamp

- What type of pie chart did Florence Nightingale invent to illustrate the causes of death in the hospitals?

    - A) Polar area diagram

- B) Donut chart

- C) Sunburst chart

- D) Radar chart

- Answer: A) Polar area diagram

- What was the name of the first nursing school that Florence Nightingale established in London in 1860?

- A) Nightingale School of Nursing

- B) St. Thomas' School of Nursing

- C) London School of Nursing

- D) Florence School of Nursing

- Answer: A) Nightingale School of Nursing

- What was the name of the bacterial infection that Florence Nightingale contracted during the Crimean War, which affected her health and mobility for most of her life?

- A) Tuberculosis

- B) Typhoid

- C) Brucellosis

- D) Cholera

- Answer: C) Brucellosis

- What was the name of the highest civilian honor that Florence Nightingale received from King Edward VII in 1907?

   - A) Order of Merit

   - B) Order of the British Empire

   - C) Order of the Bath

   - D) Order of St. Michael and St. George

   - Answer: A) Order of Merit

- What was the name of the county in England where Florence Nightingale was buried in a simple grave in the family plot, according to her wishes?

   - A) Hampshire

   - B) Somerset

   - C) Kent

   - D) Essex

   - Answer: A) Hampshire

- Interactive Activities for Kids

Hello, this is Bing. I can suggest some interactive activities for kids inspired by Florence Nightingale's life and legacy. Here are some examples:

- Make a lamp: Florence Nightingale was known as the Lady with the Lamp, because she used a lamp to light her way as she visited the patients at night. You can make your own lamp using a glass jar, a tea light candle, some wire, and some decorations. You can also write a message of hope or gratitude on a piece of paper and attach it to the jar. You can use your lamp to brighten up your room or to share some light with someone else.

- Play a matching game: Florence Nightingale was a pioneer of statistics and data visualization. She used graphs and charts to show the causes of death and the effects of her reforms in the hospitals. You can play a matching game with some of her diagrams and their explanations. You can print out some of her diagrams from the internet, such as the polar area diagram or the coxcomb chart, and cut them into pieces. You can also print out some sentences that describe what the diagrams show, and cut them into pieces.

You can then mix up the pieces and try to match the diagrams with their explanations. You can also make your own diagrams using some data that you collect or find online, and challenge someone else to match them with their explanations.

- Create a timeline: Florence Nightingale had a long and eventful life, full of challenges, adventures, and achievements. You can create a timeline of her life using some paper, a ruler, a pencil, and some markers. You can also use some stickers, photos, or drawings to illustrate the events. You can research some of the important dates and facts about her life from books, articles, or websites. You can also include some of the events that happened in the world during her lifetime, such as the Crimean War, the Industrial Revolution, or the Women's Suffrage Movement. You can use your timeline to learn more about her life and the history of her time.

- Write a letter: Florence Nightingale wrote many letters to her family, friends, colleagues, and supporters, as well as to the authorities and the public. She used her letters to share her experiences, opinions, and proposals, and to influence others to support her causes. You can write a letter to Florence Nightingale, pretending that you are one of the people who received her letters, or that you are someone who admires her work. You can use your letter to ask her some questions, to thank her for her contributions, or to tell her about your own interests and goals. You can also write a letter from Florence Nightingale to someone else, pretending that you are her, and using some of the information that you learned about her life and work. You can use your letter to explain your actions, to request some help, or to express your feelings. You can also write a letter to a nurse or a midwife who works today, and tell them how you appreciate their work and how they continue Florence Nightingale's legacy.

15. Conclusion

Florence Nightingale was a remarkable woman who dedicated her life to improving the health and well-being of people around the world. She was a pioneer of modern nursing, a visionary advocate for healthcare reforms, and an innovator of statistics and data visualization. She rose to fame during the Crimean War, where she improved the conditions and the outcomes of the military hospitals. She established the first secular and modern nursing school, and elevated the status and the standards of nursing as a profession. She also influenced the development of healthcare policies and practices, by using her reputation and evidence to lobby for her causes. She faced many challenges and obstacles, such as illness, opposition, and isolation, but she overcame them with her faith, passion, and perseverance. She left behind a legacy of nursing theory, education, and practice, as well as healthcare policies and practices, that influenced the development of nursing and healthcare around the world. She was also an inspiration and a role model for many nurses and other healthcare professionals, who followed her footsteps and continued her legacy.

We have explored some of the aspects of Florence Nightingale's life and impact, but there is much more to learn and discover about her. She was a complex and fascinating person, who had many interests and achievements, as well as many challenges and struggles. She wrote many books, reports, letters, and articles, which reveal her thoughts, feelings, and opinions on various topics and issues. She also had many relationships and interactions with different people, who influenced and supported her in different ways. She also lived in a dynamic and changing world, which shaped and challenged her in different ways. She also had a lasting and enduring impact on the world, which can still be seen and felt today.

If you are interested in learning more about Florence Nightingale, you can find many resources and opportunities to do so. You can read some of the books, articles, and websites that I have suggested, or you can search for more online or in your library. You can also visit some of the museums, monuments, and memorials dedicated to her, or you can join some of the events and activities that celebrate her. You can also talk to some of the nurses and midwives who work today, and learn how they apply her principles and practices in their work. You can also reflect on some of the values and lessons that you can learn from her life, and how you can apply them in your own life.

Florence Nightingale's life and impact are worth exploring and appreciating, as they can enrich and inspire us in many ways. She was a trailblazer in the field of nursing and healthcare, and her impact is still felt today. She was also a human being, who had her strengths and weaknesses, her joys and sorrows, her dreams and realities. She was a remarkable woman, who changed the world with her courage, kindness, and intelligence. She was Florence Nightingale, and we can learn a lot from her.

16. Additional Resources

- Recommended Books and Websites for Further Reading and Educational Materials on Florence Nightingale

If you want to learn more about Florence Nightingale's life and contributions, here are some books and websites that I recommend:

- Florence Nightingale: The Making of an Icon by Mark Bostridge[1]. This is a comprehensive and authoritative biography of Nightingale, based on extensive research and access to her private papers. It covers all aspects of her life, from her childhood and family to her work and legacy, and reveals her complex and fascinating personality.

- Florence Nightingale: A Very Brief History by Lynn McDonald[2]. This is a concise and accessible introduction to Nightingale's life and work, written by a leading scholar and editor of her collected works. It highlights her main achievements and challenges, and dispels some of the myths and misconceptions about her.

- Florence Nightingale at First Hand by Lynn McDonald[3]. This is a collection of Nightingale's own writings, selected and edited by McDonald, that illustrate her thoughts, feelings, and opinions on various topics and issues. It includes letters, reports, articles, and books, as well as some unpublished material.

- Florence Nightingale: A Reference Guide to Her Life and Works by Lynn McDonald[4]. This is a comprehensive and up-to-date reference guide to Nightingale's life and works, covering the major events, places, and people in her life, as well as her publications, correspondence, and influence. It also includes a chronology, a bibliography, and an index.

- Florence Nightingale: Nursing Pioneer by BBC Four[5]. This is a documentary film that follows the life and work of Nightingale, and shows how she revolutionized modern nursing. It features interviews with experts, historians, and nurses, as well as dramatizations and archival footage.

- The life and work of Florence Nightingale by BBC Teach[6]. This is a video clip that summarizes the life and work of Nightingale, and shows how she grew up to become a nurse during the Crimean War. It is suitable for children aged 7-11, and can be used as a teaching resource for history and citizenship.

- Florence Nightingale: Her Impact on Nursing and Colonialism by NurseJournal[7]. This is an article that examines the legacy of Nightingale, and discusses how her beliefs and actions were influenced by the colonial context of her time. It also explores how her history has been promoted through a white cultural lens, and how it can perpetuate the colonization of nursing.

- Online Learning by Florence Nightingale Foundation[8]. This is a series of online courses that aim to develop the leadership skills and potential of nurses and midwives. The courses are based on the principles and practices of Nightingale, and are designed to be innovative, engaging, and interactive.

Made in the USA
Monee, IL
05 March 2024

54480322R00066